The Cause and Cure of Breast Cancer

Dick Schuyt
Bachelors degree in Physical Education and Physical Therapy

THE CAUSE AND CURE OF BREAST CANCER
by Dick Schuyt
Copyright © 2015 by Dick Schuyt

Cover Design by: Jimi Rainier
Interior Design by: Will Rainier

15 16 17 18 19 * 98765432
Printed in the United States of America

INTRODUCTION

WHEN SOMEONE HAS fallen into shark infested water and you see that they cannot swim, the least you can do is throw 'm a floating device with a rope to pull 'm ashore.

I work as a physical therapist in home healthcare, treating people at home after a hospital stay or coming home from a surgery. After seeing so many patients struggling for their life when going through the ordeal of cancer treatment, chemo treatment and radiation, I felt I just had to share my discoveries with them.

Initially I wrote a book about the alternative treatments for cancer with the titles: "the Cancer Coach" and "Away with Cancer". I wrote it to help people fight cancer. I received a number of very encouraging letters from people who had re-found their health. But I knew that I still had not really found what I was looking for. In the back of my mind I always knew that there had to be a link between sickness and how we feel inside. Our mental and emotional inner core had to be involved somehow in the state of our physical body...

Then I read about Dr. Rijke Geert Hamer and I started studying his books and chart. As I studied his ideas about health and sickness, everything started to come together and I realized that I had found what I was looking for.

When I finished Dr. Hamer's books I applied his knowledge to my patients and, by talking to them and asking many questions, I found, to my great surprise, Dr. Hamer's theories to be right every time.

In the following years I tried to convince my patients of the truth that had become so obvious to me, but in most cases this was like telling a sinker how to swim. Too often they gave me the blank stare and I knew I had to find better ways to get through to them. For many of the people I visited at home it could mean the difference between life and death. And so it may even be for you, reading these first pages.

So here is a little booklet about breast cancer. I wrote it in kitchen table English because it is important that you understand it and then take the knowledge in this book and tell it to your loved ones and neighbors. I have not yet found a book that simply describes Dr. Hamer's theories in an understandable way to girls and women who do not have a medical background and so I felt I had to give it a shot. This book is not about fighting cancer; it's about *healing* cancer.

For this reason I did not use most of Dr. Hamer's terminology and I refrained from explaining the laws of the system of Dr. Hamer's GNM (Germanic New Medicine), since this would put an unnecessary burden on the reader who bought this book to read about the cause of breast cancer.

I hope that by reading this booklet many will become fascinated, like me, in the material that Dr. Hamer has provided in his books and chart.

Dr. Hamer's writings not only deal with cancer, but with the whole gamut of diseases. So why only write a book about breast cancer?

I chose for breast cancer since most of the principles of GNM can be easily explained while dealing with this type of cancer and a book about the whole spectrum of cancer would not fit in a lady's hand bag.

And beside this; breast cancer is rampant and is taking too many women hostage.

When women like Angelina Jolie are OK with having their breasts 'amputated' out of fear of contracting breast cancer somewhere in their life, we have come to a crisis in the medical care of women. We're not winning the war on cancer and we can't rely on our government, which is in cahoots with the multinational pharmaceutical corporations, to come with real answers.

Even President Barak Hussein Obama broke his promise to us when he looked us in the eyes and told us we could keep our doctor if we liked him or her.

Many women are afraid, bewildered and in panic. That's why this book is necessary! It will show you what causes the cancer in your breasts and how to save them.

I say: *when you like your breast you can keep 'em!*

DISCLAIMER

The statements in this book have not been evaluated by the Food and Drug Administration. This book is written with the intend to educate people about a vision on healthcare not widely known.

The author of this book is *not* a medical doctor and not qualified, does not want and does not mean to prescribe any treatment, medication or supplement.

You are advised to consult an open minded health-care professional before choosing any route in your search for health.

The author does not warrant that the information contained in this book is in every respect accurate or complete and he is not responsible, nor liable for any errors or omissions that may be found in this book, or for the results obtained from the use of such information.

This book simply is an attempt to report about a doctor who has claimed and proven to have found a way to successfully heal cancer.

I just report his findings. You decide!

ONE

CANCER IN AMERICA

AS A MEDICAL professional, working in the Home Healthcare setting, I meet women who have active breast cancer, or who have survived it. And, although it is not really my business, when they open up about their illness, I ask them the question: -"*do you know why you have cancer?*"- After a puzzled look I always get the same answer: -"well..., *I don't know, I guess I never really thought about that!*"-

For my inquisitive nature this is like screeching your fingernails over the chalkboard! However, I think I understand their answer. In our western mindset we have learned to believe that the doctor, or the medical professional, is the authority in our life who has been trained to take care of all our physical troubles. He, or she, has the knowledge to oversee the vast ocean of different diseases, ailments and conditions that people may be suffering from and only he / she is, by law, allowed to choose, inform you about, and prescribe a certain treatment.

We have learned to accept that reality and most of us will not bring up the question of the *cause* of our disease in the short time that is given us in the face to face time with '*our*' doctor.

And even when we would ask the question, our doctor would not be able to tell us more than is published in his yearly updated desk reference, which tells us basically that the cause of cancer is unknown.

He or she will tell you about the different medications and treatment options, different cancer centers, oncologists (= cancer-doctors) and specialists who will assist you in the treatment of your particular cancer. But the cause of cancer is unknown, which should make you pretty suspicious of their proposed treatment.

How can you successfully treat a disease while you have no idea as to how it originates and what the cause is? Hmmmm...!

However, here comes the true nature of the word treatment into focus. Treatment is not a cure. Treatment does not pretend to eliminate the disease or condition. Treatment is designed to find and push down the symptoms, the bleeding, the pain, the inflammation, by medications, or it may restore function in an arthritic joint by replacing it with a metal joint through surgery.

Chemo treatment, radiation, surgery, medications, biopsies, mammo-grams, X-rays, breast implants, are all part of the *treatment plan* for cancer. Chemo treatment is the treatment of choice. An article in the prestigious 'Journal of Clinical Oncology', that covers a 12 year study of the effect of chemo-treatment, shows that chemo-treatment has a success rate of 3%! It fails 97 out of 100!

In an interview, Dr. Peter Glidden, BS and ND, author of the book *'The MD Emperor has no clothes'*, goes on record and says: - *"The only reason chemo-treatment is used is because doctors make money from it."* -

And: - *"With chemo-treatment the prescribing doctor gets a (financial) cut-out."* -

In the October 2014 issue of 'Life-extension' magazine, William Faloon writes in the article called 'As we see it': - *"... 'managed care' has diluted the quality of care provided by many oncologists. In a stunning new development, a health insurance company is offering oncologists $ 350.- per month for each patient that is put on the company's recommended regimen."* -

You guessed it; the **recommended regimen** is the list with the cheapest and least effective medicines.

If the oncologist keeps his or her prescriptions within the recommended protocol of the insurance company, the financial incentive that is pocketed by the end of the year is $4200.- per patient!

Since President Nixon initialized the "war on cancer" we still do not know what causes cancer. And for the cancer industry it is important that this horrible situation stays just the way it is. This industry is monopolized by enormous corporations with very deep pockets. Pharmaceutical corporations, with billions of dollars in yearly turnover, are driven by shareholders who demand profit. Profit is found only in treatment. Any CEO of a pharma-comp knows that and will stimulate his lab-workers and technicians to come up with the latest drug, the best imaging equipment, mammogram machine and what have you.

One thing they will stay away from. One thing will kill their business, profit, and livelihood. It will bring stockholders to fury and will bring the pharma business to death's door.

What is that? It is a... **cure for cancer**...!

The betrayal of the American people by the American Medical Association, the Cancer Societies, the insurance companies and the justice system is well documented. Doctors who found ways to cure cancer were taken to court, jailed, locked up for years, killed, their work destroyed or simply ignored. Many have escaped the country, practicing in Mexico or South America. This little book will not deal with all of this.

In this dis-functional medical culture there is no cure for cancer, the cause of cancer is unknown and it is kept in the unknown for corporate welfare. It is the sad result of predatory capitalism and the end of it is not in sight. Corporatism and politics are geared towards taking over the world to have control over everything and everybody, and the medical establishment has become instrumental in the quest to control the populace of the nations.

Even worse; the societies that are focused on creating this one world control over the populations of the world have openly expressed their desire to find ways to *reduce* the number of people living on the earth. To them cancer and heart disease are to remain the inescapable and legitimate killers in our Western culture, 'naturally' regulating the number of the populace. A very sinister truth!

But enough about this. It is just to show you that you're on your own, Kiddo, and I am glad you turned to this booklet to find what you are looking for: an answer to your question -*"Why do I, or my loved one have cancer? What caused it?"*- And there *is* an answer!

Two

CANCER TREATMENT IN THE 21ST CENTURY

Imagine for a moment that you sit on the couch, watching your favorite TV program all by yourself with the cat purring on your lap. Suddenly you notice that water is slowly covering the floor of your room. So you pull up your feet and put the cat on the couch, you walk over to the kitchen and grab some pans and a bucket and start scooping up the water and fill the bucket. You empty the bucket in the kitchen sink and run back to the living room, but then you realize that you are smarter than that and you pull the vacuum from the wall in the closet. After plugging it in, the vacuum is filled in no time and shorts out. Now what! Water is rising! Yes, you have another great idea: towels, lots of towels. No, forget the towels; there is too much water already. Stop, try to think. Water, floor, flowing, rising, OK I got it! Since the water flows down from the stairs you build a dam!! Of course, a dam! And you manage to push the couch against the first steps of the stairs. Great idea! Now you can call 911. When the police arrive they all grab towels, pans, buckets and help out as well as they can. Then the dam breaks and the water flushing you out with the furniture and the police into the street…

Need I go on?

Now, of course this will never happen to you, because you will immediately realize that you left the water running of the bath that you were filling upstairs, you'll run up the stairs and close the tap! And all the other decisions mentioned above that were made to get rid of the water were simply very in-practical and dysfunctional. When you saw the water coming down the stairs you knew right away what the cause was and you acted fast and adequately.

You dealt with the CAUSE of the problem!

There was nothing wrong with the water, but it appeared at the wrong place and with too much volume. Although you meant to use the water to your benefit to enjoy a relaxing hot bath with candle light, you simply forgot the bath and you were too late closing the tap.

I am sad to say that the comedy-caper situation you just read can be applied to the moment where cancer starts happening in someone's life. There is fear, panic, wrong decisions, poor advice, all sorts of 'treatments', doctors, hospitals, cancer centers and what not. But no one is seriously asking the right question of where the water is coming from, or: what the cause of cancer is.

Now, you'll say "*now wait a minute; my doctor is very serious about my physical wellbeing and I have a good relationship with him...*".

That may be so, but realize that your doctor, specialist, or oncologist doesn't know and doesn't ask about the cause of cancer. And to their defense we can say that each of these medical professionals will lose their license if any of them does not follow the 'golden rule'. This rule is also known as '*consensus medicine*'.

It means that doctors have to practice medicine according to the rules set in stone by the American Medical Association (AMA). Doctors have to do what their peers are practicing, which means: there is no place for any alternative medicine. When doctors step out of line they lose their license and their livelihood and have to close their office.

But even if your doctor would go over and beyond the limits that have been set for him, how will he help you if he does not know the cause of cancer?

The Newsweek cover of March 2014 read:

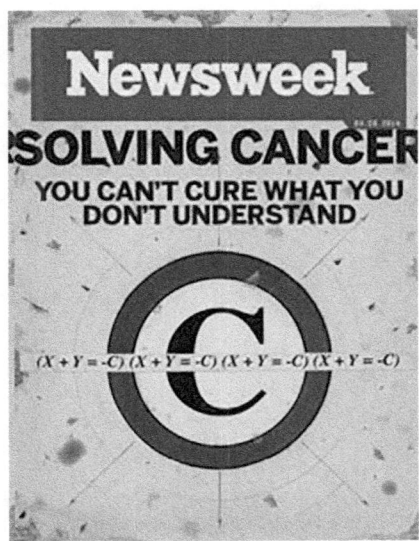

So how, pray tell, can you even start to treat cancer effectively while you don't even know the cause of it!

This is where we are now: there is treatment and treatment and more treatment, but the cause of cancer is not really being looked at or studied. Like in the analogy of the water running down the stairs, treatment is like using pots and pans and towels to keep the water from taking over the house. And although there is a lot of talk about cancer, hardly anyone is talking about the water-tap that is open.

Yes, billions of dollars are being spent in research, but the research is not aimed at finding a cure for cancer. It is aimed at developing new pills, or a new technology, or **anything that promises profit.**

Again; the cause of cancer is not being looked at because when you find the cause, you'll find the cure and that is very counter-productive from a business standpoint.

This book is an attempt to show you where the water tap is and how to close it.

THREE

FINDING THE CAUSE OF CANCER

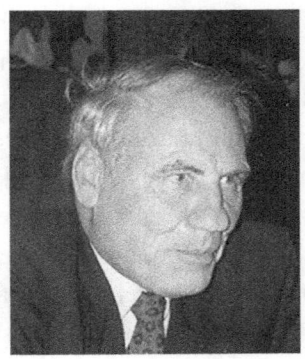

I WANT TO INTRODUCE you to a medical doctor who did find the cause of cancer and who spent the rest of his life trying to treat and educate people, although the medical establishment tried to keep that from happening with literally every means possible. If any man has fought for you to be informed about the true nature and cause of cancer it is Dr. Rijke Geerd Hamer, born in 1935.

Dr. Hamer studied medicine and theology in Tuebingen in Germany. His inventions enabled him to move to Italy and work amongst the poor in the slums of Rome, free of charge. While in Rome in 1978, his son was accidentally shot and died in his arms a little later. Soon after this horrible experience Dr. Hamer, who never had any serious illness, found himself to have testicular cancer. He theorized that the testicular cancer could be related to the sudden death of his son. Growing a tumor in the one male organ pertaining to procreation, while grieving for a dead son, aroused his attention. Could it be that his cancer somehow was triggered by his emotional turmoil and his mourning?

In the following years Dr. Hamer studied about the possible truth of his theory. He talked with his patients and re-read the case histories of thousands of his patients. He examined thousands of brain scans and what he found was well worth his time and effort. He discovered that every patient suffering from cancer in the body had a swelling in the brain that could be clearly seen and identified on the brain scans as concentric circles; a "target-mark" encircling the particular area in the brain that was involved with the particular cancer in the body. Patients with stomach cancer had a target mark around the area of the brain dealing with the stomach and those with breast cancer had target marks around the brain-area directing the breast, etc.

He also found that cancer in his patients always started right after a sudden and unexpected, emotional shock and that after the shock the target mark became visible on the brain scan.

While working on all this Dr. Hamer's testicular tumor stopped growing and slowly, over time, disappeared all by itself. It appeared that his tumor stopped growing after his initial grief for his son had subsided. And through this horrible experience and his research Dr. Hamer had learned the following: cancer happens after a sudden, unexpected emotional shock to the system, after which the brain starts to swell in the certain area that connects to the part of the body where the cancer starts to develop.

He realized that he had found the cause of his cancer.

The enormous tragedy of Dr. Hamer's son Dirk, dying in his arms, had somehow triggered his bio-system to start a tumor process in his testicle, growing more seed-producing cells and tissue in the testicle. It seemed as if his biological system tried to... *help him*... by increasing the production of semen to make up for the loss of his offspring. The emotional shock of his son's death had triggered his bio-system to...come to his rescue.

In the following years Dr. Hamer tried out his new theory of cancer on his patients with tremendous results. Instead of the usual treatment with chemicals or radiation Dr. Hamer took the time with every patient to talk and find out if the patient had a possible psychological shock. He also ordered brain scans to be taken of all of them. The outcomes were unmistakable. Every cancer was precipitated by an emotional shock or conflict and the brain scans always showed the target marks in the involved area.

Through years of further study Dr. Hamer managed to chart the different cancers, connecting every type of cancer with its own typical emotional shock or conflict. Skin cancer was related to *separation conflicts*, lung cancer to *death fright*, bone cancer to *self-devaluation conflicts*, etc., etc.

He treated every patient by taking time to talk extensively with him or her, going back in time with them to find the moment of impact of the emotional shock. He examined the brain-scans and talked and helped the patient towards his or her resolution of their emotional conflict or shock. No chemo treatment, radiation or surgery. But with all of them their cancer process took a turn for the better after they came to resolution of their conflicts or shocks. Tumors would stop growing and die off, slowly to be re-absorbed by the body system itself.

Dr. Hamer condensed all his knowledge in a medical system that he called Germanic New Medicine (GNM). It is necessary to highlight a few of the principles and dynamics described in GNM that will help us to better understand Dr. Hamer's ideas and perspective of cancer and of disease in general.

FOUR

WHAT IS CANCER?

THE INTERNET ENCYCLOPEDIA: 'Wikipedia' defines cancer as –*"a broad group of diseases involving unregulated cell growth"*-. When we think of 'unregulated growth' we think of more cells, or less cells, or a speeding up, or a slowing down of cell growth. So, speaking of cancer, we distinguish two dynamics: the growth (multiplication, or proliferation) of cells that we find in tumors and the decrease of cells (cell death or necrotizing of cells) that we find in the 'holes' appearing as bone cancer.

And somehow the growth and the death of cells is unregulated, which means so much as; things are not going according to plan, or there is no plan, direction, or proper management of the cell growth / death.

Unregulated cell growth sounds like chaos, directionless, meaningless, or diseased. It leaves us the impression that our body is extremely vulnerable and easily dis-regulated, prone to mistakes, difficult to defend, with random illness and easily overcome by unknown enemies.

We will find in the next chapters that this is all in great contrast with Dr. Hamer's Germanic New Medicine.

In GNM, diseases are called "special meaningful biological programs of nature", that are designed to benefit us and help us in our daily lives. Cancer too, in GNM, is a meaningful program with the purpose of properly and functionally responding in a physical way to a psychological, or better: emotional jolt to our system. Although in the medical world cancer is seen as an enemy that we have to wage war against, you will find in the following pages that, in GNM, the cancer process has a very special purpose, programmed into our nature, to aid and assist us in the challenges of life and to simply help us to survive.

THE TWO DIFFERENT WAYS CANCER CAN MANIFEST.

Healing is the body's way of repairing what is broke. We all can agree on that.

Let's look a bit closer at what happens when healing takes place in the body.

When the city started work on a broken water pipe in our county, traffic was rerouted for almost a month, and from a distance we could see the development of the work. There was a coming and going of trucks loaded with dirt and equipment, hauling dirt away from the site during the excavation process. And three weeks later dirt was hauled back to the site to cover up the new pipe and to fix the road.

In our body a similar dynamic takes place; for some repair we, initially, need more tissue, or more cells, more connective tissue or bone tissue, while in other situations we need to start with taking tissue away from the repair site.

When a bone breaks the body immediately starts a repair process, first the old bone and tissue that was damaged is taken away and when the site is cleaned up and repaired new bone is filled in, in just the right places and eventually the bone is healed and even stronger than before.

More tissue is of course established when the body system orders the growth and multiplication of cells that form tissue.

Less tissue we get when tissue cells are ordered to die and disintegrate and the dead residue is taken away by the white blood cells that are the garbage men of the body.

This process of directed cell death is called apoptosis, or necrosis. When a splinter has pierced the skin of the finger, the body orders the cells around the splinter to die so that a wound bed with puss forms around the splinter. Now, with a little squeezing the splinter can fairly easily be pushed out of the skin. The little wound that is left we call an ulcer. After the puss and the dead cells are squeezed out, the little wound heals by the growth of new cells at the place where cells had died.

So, both cell growth as well as cell death play a very important and functional role in the maintenance of our health.

Both these processes are directed by the brain and the brain in turn is directed by the psyche, by the way we feel and think.

Or to turn it around: our psyche has a direct benevolent and meaningful influence in the physical processes of our physical body! The way we think and feel is directly translated into our physical body and the body reacts by an increase or a decrease of cells and tissue in a certain place.

This dynamic is happening continually and everywhere in the body, maintaining the balance for good health and for meaningful adjustments to the challenges that life offers us. Like a beautiful concert played by an orchestra and directed by the director, with moments of almost silence but then again interrupted by crescendos. Up and down, high and low, more cells, less cells, tissue growth and tissue death.

In the following pages you will see that, although cancer has been given a bad press, it too is part of this symphony of life and it too is a **meaningful biological program** with a purpose to benefit, assist and heal the body.

So why has cancer become such a terrorist?

Let me explain. The trouble starts when these programs, that were started up to our benefit and healing, **continue their action for too long** and are not directed to stop.

When you cook milk you have to switch off the gas at just the right time or you have a big clean up to do. Or when you pour concrete for a floor and you let the truck driver pour for too long, you are in a lot of trouble. Although cooking milk and pouring concrete are very meaningful things to do, you'll be in a great deal of trouble **when you do not stop in time.**

When, for instance, the multiplication and growth of breast tissue cells is not stopped at the right time, a lump will form, which we call a tumor or a cancer.

Or when properly directed cell death is not stopped in time, we'll end up with an ulcer or even a hole in the tissue.

So the duration of these processes is of the essence!

The trouble of cancer starts when healing isn't stopped at the right time because the psyche continues to order the healing process to go on.

In Dr. Hamer's cancer case; the new growth of testicular cells was meant for his wellbeing and it started right after the loss of his son. But because his severe and prolonged grief, his psyche kept directing the brain to continue making testicular cells up to a point where cells kept piling up and a tumor was forming. And then it was diagnosed as...cancer!

Through this experience Dr. Hamer found that the cause of his cancer was his continued grief process.

If his grieving had lasted only for a week he would never have noticed the process that was going on in his testicle.

He had learned from his own body that his feelings and emotions were the initial cause of his cancer.

He also found that his cancer had stopped growing after he had come to resolution of his grieving.

And that was the onset of his further discoveries that we will talk about in the following chapters.

FIVE

THE TWO DIFFERENT PHASES IN CANCER.

Dr. Hamer also found that cancer always runs its course in two different and identifiable phases. He called these two phases; the **conflict active phase** and the **healing phase**.

In the first phase we see the development of cancer until the patient has come to resolution of the conflict, the worry or the fear. That is the time the cancer stops and the healing sets in.

THE CONFLICT ACTIVE PHASE

The conflict active phase starts right at the time of the sudden emotional conflict, fright, or shock.

The patient is in a kind of nervous state with cold hands and feet, poor appetite, difficulty sleeping and waking up early, immediately being reminded by the worry, or fear, or shock.

It is like the bio-system is forcing the patient to become aware of the shock, or worry, in order to start the process of coming to resolution of the emotions as soon as possible.

When taking a brain scan, a few concentric circles like a target mark can now be seen around the area in the brain where the cell growth or the cell death is being directed. The location in the brain is directly related to the body part where the cancer starts.

(This is hard evidence of the truth of Dr.'Hamer's approach to cancer, which can clearly be seen by a trained eye and cannot be reasoned away.)

Meanwhile, when the shock in the psyche triggers a program that demands cell growth, the tissue, overtime, can develop into tumor, growing slow or fast, dependent on the intensity of the experienced conflict or shock. The more intense the shock is experienced the faster and more aggressive the tumor grows. The less intense conflict produces a slower growing tumor.

When the emotional shock starts a program in the brain that directs cell death, the tissue, overtime, can develop into an ulcer. Here too it is the intensity of the perceived shock that determines the speed and extent of the cell death and the ulceration process.

THE HEALING PHASE

The second phase, or healing phase, starts after the person has come to resolution of his or her conflict / shock. When this happens the patient can sleep again, his or her worry is over, the fear is gone, or the shock subsided. Hands and feet are warm again. No more arousal of the emotions. There is tiredness during the day with the patient wanting to rest and sleep at odd times. There may be a raise in body temperature and the appetite has returned.

The target mark on the brain scan will slowly fade away.

The cell multiplication or cell death that was ordered by the psyche, will now stop. Where there was cell growth and perhaps a tumor, now this cell mass will be directed to die and be gobbled up by micro-organisms that are provided by the body itself.

Where there was cell death with ulceration, maybe to the extent of a hole in the tissue, there will now be a clean-up by the body and new cell growth to fill in the hole that has been created by the (prolonged) cell death.

In the healing phase the damage that was done in the conflict active phase is stopped, cleaned up and reversed. The tumors are removed and the holes are replenished with new tissue. And although this healing phase can be messy, with pain, swelling, puss, bacteria's (the clean-up crew) and a temperature, when it is completed, the patient has a restored body.

(The clean-up crew, we talked about, consists of micro-organisms, like bacteria and fungi. In the conflict active phase the body already starts to breed these bacteria and/or fungi in anticipation of the need for clean up in the healing phase. This is one of the great wonders of our body!)

That is pretty good news, right?!

So, now we not only have found the cause of cancer, but we also have seen how cancer is stopped and how our own body cleans up the cancer mess over time! This is fantastic news and it should be in the headlines of every newspaper for weeks to come!

TWO SHORT CASE STUDIES:

Marjory (an old patient of mine) lived in with her daughter Jill, who was an alcoholic. Every day Marjory experienced her daughter getting drunk and abusive around lunch time. She could not talk with her because Jill would get angry and Marjory was afraid Jill would kick her out of the house. Marjory needed the cheap room and board from Jill and so their lives were intertwined. Marjory worried day and night about the health of her only daughter. When I started treating Marjory for knee problems she told me she had stage 4 breast cancer. I could share with her the ideas of Doctor Hamer; that her cancer was caused by her continued worry for her daughter, and she believed this to be the case. But Marjory could not get to resolution of her worry problem, being confronted daily with her daughter's drinking problem. She could not talk with her daughter and three months later she died while going through extensive Chemo treatment.

(Marjory had been in the cancer active phase for a long time; too long. The intensity of her worry was high due to the daily drunkenness and abusive behavior by her daughter. Her cancer

therefore was aggressive and fast growing. She could not resolve her worrying and so she never reached the healing phase of cancer. It was not the cancer that killed her, but the treatment.)

Here is another one.

Jenny comes home from the doctor and with tears in her eyes she calls her friend Trish, blurting out: *"my doctor found a lump in my breast ..!"* Trish tells her: *"stay where you are, I'll be right over!"* They sit at the kitchen table with coffee and a box of Kleenex. Trish has some understanding of Dr. Hamer's ideas of the treatment of cancer and asks Jill to go back in time and tell her what happened in the period when, according to the doctor, the cancer started. Jill remembers her terrible worry when she heard that Tim her husband, who is stationed in Iraq, had taken a bullet in his chest. She could not stop worrying and woke up every morning since then with great anxiety. Trish understands that Jenny has to let go of her worry and anguish to stop the cancer from growing and decides to visit her every morning after the kids leave for school. After much talking, praying, crying and laughing and realizing that her husband is OK, Jenny hears at her next doctor's visit that the 'lump' in her breast has not grown any larger... Her cancer active phase has finished, she is in the healing phase and the cell growth has stopped.

(Jenny was blessed to have a friend who could explain to her that her cancer was triggered by an emotional shock or worry. Trish proved to be a great friend and stayed with Jenny until she could let her worries go and could come to resolution. Jenny transferred into the healing phase of cancer where the tumor (the lump) died off and could be absorbed by the body.)

Two case stories where the difference of outcome clearly is found in whether one comes to resolution of the worry, or shock, or not. It can mean the difference between life and death.

Now, before we start talking about breast cancer, we need to know one more principle used in GNM that will help you greatly in identifying the cause of breast cancer. Handedness!

Six

HANDEDNESS

One great tool that I have learned from Dr. Hamer is the principle of "handedness". I use it every time in my physical therapy practice when I evaluate a new patient.

As you know, our brain is divided into two halves. There is a creative brain half and a more mathematical half. It has been the subject of many jokes.

Dr. Hamer found that there is another difference that is extremely valuable for us to know and which gives us better understanding in the influence of our emotions on our biological system. He called it: "*handedness*", or: being right, or left handed.

When you are right handed your left body side is your "nest" side and your right body side is your "partner" side. Any condition or disease that manifests on the left side of your body can be related to your "*nest*", or to who or whatever is in your "nest". (Your children, a mother you may take care of, your pet, or favorite doll, etc.) When things manifest in the right side of your body they are related to your partner or spouse, a good friend or a colleague you work with.

When you are left handed it is just the opposite way. Problems on your left side will relate to your spouse or a friend, or colleague and ailments manifesting on your right side have to do with your 'nest' and anyone that is in it.

When you are or have been a Mom, you know this to be true: when feeding your child you carry the child in your left arm when you are right handed. This frees up your right hand to hold the bottle, or adjust the diaper, or hold the phone. You left handed Moms like to keep your left hand free for these things. It simply is a thing of nature.

Some folks do not know what their dominant side is. They are ambidextrous and can write with their right hand and paint with their left, for instance. There is however a way to find out what your dominant side is: just clap your hands and the hand that is on top is your dominant hand.

Since breasts always come in sets of two, a left and a right, this handedness tool will give us very important information about the specific cause of breast cancer.

Now before we dive into the real meat of the book, let's do a quick review on the important aspects of GNM that we've found so far.

Review:

- ✓ The conflict active phase of cancer starts after a sudden shock conflict, fright, or worry that takes one completely by surprise.
- ✓ The psyche that is affected by the emotional turmoil somehow chooses a plan of action and directs the brain to a meaningful, physical response.
- ✓ This response relates to a certain place in the body, a particular tissue.
- ✓ On a brain scan a "target mark" can now be seen around the brain area relating to the location of this tissue in the body.
- ✓ The conflict active phase manifests either by cell growth (tumor), or by cell death (ulcer) in the tissue.
- ✓ When the resolution of the conflict takes too long, the lump (or tumor), or the ulcer continue to develop and eventually is found by the patient of by the doctor and diagnosed as cancer.
- ✓ When there is resolution of the shock, worry or conflict, the cancer process stops and now the healing phase begins; the tumor or ulcer is cleaned up by the body.
- ✓ The healing phase takes twice as long as the conflict active phase and in this phase everything is being reversed and restored. Hallelujah!

Seven

BREAST CANCER

Now, BEFORE WE start dealing with cancer of the breasts, let's take a moment to refresh our knowledge of the normal functioning of the breasts.

Functionally speaking, breasts are those parts of a female body that can provide nutrition to a new born baby or young child. The milk glands contain tissues that produce milk and the milk ducts enable the transport of milk from the glands to the nipple and thus to the baby's mouth (see diagram on next page).

During the last months of pregnancy the milk production is started; the glands make milk that flows into the ducts where milk accumulates and is transported to the nipple and to be sucked out by the newborn. This milk production can last even for years, but eventually will stop and everything will turn back to how it was before the pregnancy.

Of course there are all the other tissues that enable the production and transport of milk, like blood vessels, lymph vessels and nodes, fatty tissue and different supportive tissues. But, when we talk about breast cancer it manifests mainly in two different kinds of tissues: *'glandular cancer'* in the milk glands of the breast, and *'ductal cancer'* in the milk ducts of the breast.

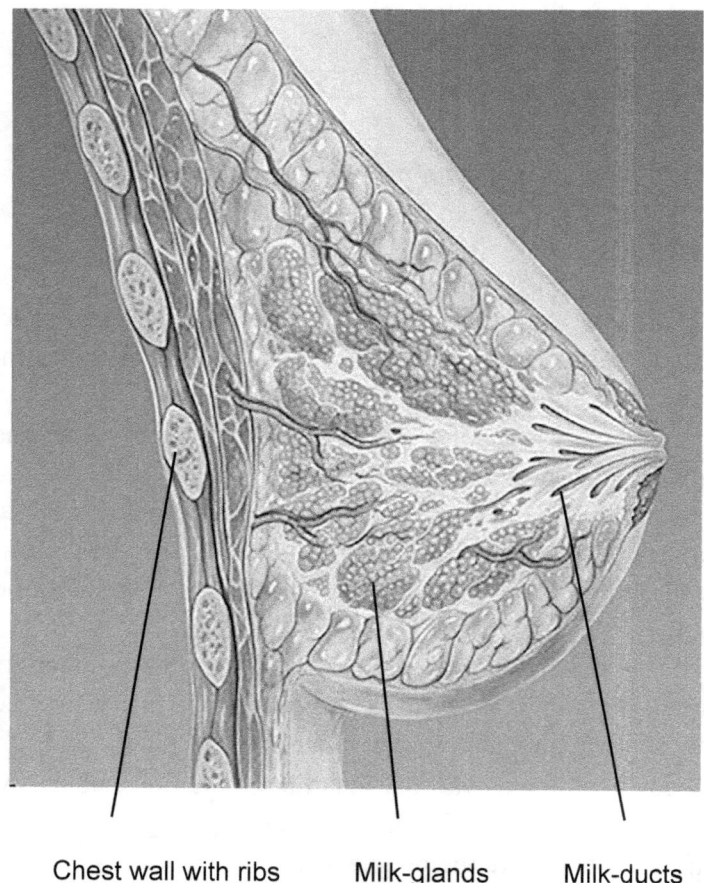

Chest wall with ribs   Milk-glands   Milk-ducts

In this picture you can see the milk glands and the milk ducts.

So, let's see what happens in the breasts when cancer appears on the scene.

EIGHT

THE CONFLICT ACTIVE PHASE OF BREAST CANCER.

W<small>E'LL DISCUSS EACH</small> type of cancer individually; we'll start with:

GLANDULAR CANCER

Glandular cancer (or glandular mammary carcinoma) is the rapid multiplication and accumulation of milk producing cells in one or more places in the breast. There is great activity going on and cells that resemble very much the glandular cells start multiplying as if there is a great need for milk. When this process is not stopped but carries on for weeks and months there will be a great pile up of glandular cells and that is what is called a 'tumor', or in English: a lump.

This cancer process starts by a sudden worry, an emotional jolt that takes the person completely by surprise. An enormous overwhelming feeling of uncertainty that can best be characterized by one word: **worry**! For instance: a loved one is unexpectedly diagnosed with a dreadful disease. A husband has not come home from work. A child is missing. Your child has a high fever and there is no doctor around. Etc., Etc. Or there may be a **serious argument** going on between the woman and someone in her nest.

The worry triggers the woman's brain into a nurturing response. It does this by directing the glandular cells in the breast to start multiplying and to get ready for the production of milk. A seemingly strange response since there is no baby, but it is nature's best way of responding to the worry. In nature, milk, or nutrition, is the richest care a female can provide when there is reason to worry.

So glandular cells are accumulating in the breast and as time progresses lumps are being formed and lumps grow into tumors. The tumors grow faster when the worry is intense or slower when it is less intense. The feeling of a little lump in the breast may be a first indication that something is wrong.

In a right handed woman who worries about a husband or good friend the lumps are found in her right breast. (handedness!)

A right handed woman who worries about a child, or her mother who lives in with her, or a pet (who all are part of her "nest"), will have the cancer growing in her left breast. (handedness!)

And of course this is all reversed for a left handed woman. She will have left breast cancer worrying for her partner and right breast cancer worrying for whoever is in her "nest".

From here the development of the cancer can go in two directions. When the woman can stop her worrying and can come to resolution of her worry conflict, the cancer will stop growing and she will enter into the healing phase of cancer. When the emotional shock has calmed down, the brain will stop directing the breast to make more glandular cells.

However, when she continues to worry and cannot stop her anxiety about the issue, the cancer process will continue and tumors will grow larger.

DUCTAL CANCER

Here too, the conflict active phase of the cancer process starts with a sudden emotional conflict, but not with a 'worry-conflict' as with glandular cancer. Ductal cancer (or intra ductal carcinoma) begins after a "**separation conflict**". Imagine a husband leaving and threatening with a divorce, or a child having left for college, leaving the parent with an empty feeling. These are situations that can lead to severe conflicts. However, do not underestimate the seemingly 'small' conflicts that can still trigger major emotional reactions in a woman, like the loss of a pet, a dear friend who is moving to another state, or even the loss of a favorite doll. All these can cause tremendous anxiety in the woman's emotional center and can become the cause of 'ductal cancer'.

There is a significant relation between ductal breast cancers and women who have had an abortion. Even years after the actual abortion, a woman can still suddenly be overcome by the realization of the separation with her aborted child.

The 'separation conflict' ignites the brain to direct the cells of the inner lining of the ducts to die. When these cells, on the inside of the ducts, die off and are drained off you can imagine that this leaves more space for milk to flow since there is now a wider opening. In nature the sudden loss of a child will immediately cause this same response in many animals.

The meaning of this response can be seen when we imagine a young to be ripped from the female's breast and to be separated from her. The sudden separation discontinues the normal drainage of milk from the breast, leaving the female / woman in a painful situation, where milk can pile up in the breast, causing all sorts of complications. There is a great need to get rid of the abundance of milk, and fast. This is why the ductal openings need to be widened quickly.

Here too, the rule of 'handedness' plays an important role: the right handed woman will have ductal cancer in the right breast suffering from a separation conflict relating to her partner, or a good friend, or colleague. The left breast will be involved when the conflict relates to her 'nest' and to those who she perceives to be in it.

For the left handed woman it is the opposite way.

When the separation conflict is not resolved in time the cell death will continue not only in the lining, but now also deeper in the walls of the ducts, causing holes in the walls and ulceration. However, when there is conflict resolution, the cell death (= cancer) will stop and the woman transfers into the healing phase, where the dead tissue will be removed by microbes and new tissue will start growing to replenish the loss of tissue in the ducts.

Later we'll talk some more about how to help someone to come to resolution of these conflicts.

RECOGNIZING THE CONFLICT ACTIVE PHASE.

So, how do you know if you or a loved one is in the conflict active phase? Most people won't notice it when they go through the beginning stage of cancer, or maybe we should say: they do not *recognize* it.

Here are some signs and symptoms we can experience in the cancer active phase.

At the moment of impact of the emotional shock, our nervous system switches over to a simpatico-tonic state where there is great awareness of the worry or the conflict, with difficulty sleeping and the subject of the conflict being constantly on our mind. Waking up early in the morning, with our conflict or worry immediately in focus and asking for attention. There is restriction of blood flow in our extremities, causing cold hands and feet, with shivering. The patient has poor appetite and there may be a raised blood pressure.

There is no fever or swelling and in most cases there is no pain, except with glandular cancer. The lump can be felt as it is developing. Stepping back for a moment and looking at these, we may see that during this phase it seems like our 'spirit + body system' is forcing us to become aware and acknowledge that something is wrong. We are kept from sleeping, we are kept in an uncomfortable state of being, we don't have an appetite, and we have the shivers, with cold hands and feet.

It is as if our system is prompting us to realize that something is wrong and we'd better get serious about it.

When we look carefully at all that is going on in the conflict active phase we could conclude that our spirit or psyche, after being aroused, warns the brain that something is wrong and that something needs to be done about it.

A choice is made then and a surprisingly functional physical response is being triggered in the body to grow tissue or to withdraw tissue. It is almost as if the psyche or the brain, or wherever the decision is made, thumbs through a huge file of 'blue-prints' and picks one program that is most appropriate to respond physically to the specific emotional conflict or worry.

What a fantastic design! What a wonderful creation! Isn't it astounding to find that the processes we call diseases in reality are programs that are there to help us to respond to the challenges that life throws at us 24/7 and 365?! If only we learn to switch off the emotional conflict or worry and the accompanying feelings at the proper time, we will never see cancer and we will be able to prevent it from ever happening!

If we can live our life with our emotional brain *'wiped clean'* on a daily or even on a weekly base, cancer will never be able to develop in our tissues.

NINE

THE HEALING PHASE OF BREAST CANCER.

AFTER RESOLUTION OF the emotional shock, fear, or worry, the healing phase starts. We see a reversal of the biological processes that happened in the cancer *active* phase.

GLANDULAR CANCER

Where **glandular tissue** grew into a tumor, we now see a stop on the multiplication of glandular cells and a dying off of the cells that formed the tumor. This process is called the necrotizing of cells, or simply: cell death. The tumor cells die and the decomposed remains of the cells are eaten and gobbled up by micro- organisms (like fungi, or bacteria). As we have seen, these micro-organisms were produced by the body already during the cancer active phase in anticipation of the necessary clean up in the future.

What a beautiful and great system!

HOWEVER! OFTEN, DUE to the discomfort experienced in the healing phase, the woman goes and sees her doctor. When the lump is detected on the mammo-gram or X-ray and the doctor starts treating with chemo treatment, radiation and / or antibiotics, the normal clean-up of dead tissue is interrupted, because the clean-up crew is... 'killed' by these chemicals and medical procedures.

In this case, the body will encapsulate the old and dead tumor with a shell of calcium and that will be the end of that! These calcium 'capsules' will always light up on an X-ray, but they are harmless, they are just old and dead tumors that were never properly cleaned up.

It is more desirable then to let the body have its own way during the healing phase so there can be a complete clean-up and restoration of the involved tissues.

DUCTAL CANCER

When a **ductal cancer** transfers into the healing phase, the cell death (the ulceration of the tissue) is stopped and the dead cells are being cleaned up, leaving a hole or cavity that needs to be filled up again with normal, healthy ductal tissue. These dead cells and the puss and 'gunk' are being drained away from the clean-up site to the outside through the nipple. This often is a painful process, especially when there is swelling at the 'job site' taking place.

Healing always goes together with swelling of the tissue and of the neighboring tissues because the healing agents are being transported to the job-site by...fluids. This swelling can cause obstruction of the ductal system itself which makes it more difficult to drain the puss away. It may be good here to try and 'milk' or massage the breast to help the puss come out.

When a ductal cancer had the chance to develop for a long time there may be so much swelling and so little drainage that the clean-up crew has to force itself a passage way to the outer skin of the breast to drain the puss away. This would of course cause a skin wound that has to be taken care of and kept clean. The body can handle all this, although it may take a good while to completely heal from all this. As said before, the healing phase often takes twice as long as the cancer active phase, but eventually there is healing of the ductal system although there may be considerable scar tissue left in the breast.

RECOGNIZING THE HEALING PHASE OF CANCER

So how do we know that we have moved into the healing phase of cancer?

As we have seen, the cancer process is stopped after the conflict or worry has been resolved. On the brain scan the 'target mark' can now be seen fading away, indicating that the swelling in the brain area is decreasing. The nervous system switches over into a vagotonic state: cold hands and feet are gone; now the patient feels warm again. There may be swelling, redness, a temperature and pain. And since the conflict has been resolved, the mind is free again to focus on other things. The patient has need of much sleep, also during the day time. A diet rich in proteins will help the patient to make healthy new tissue.

In cases that have lingered on there may be puss and stink and wounds but with all this it is good to remind ourselves that we are in the healing phase and that all this will eventually pass away and we will be cleaned up and healed.

(In the past I have tested many patients' saliva with the Litmus test to test for acidity, and I always found cancer patients to be very acid with a score of 5.0 or less. Since I am now familiar with Dr. Hamer's theories, I better understand why this is. When the body is cleaning up cancer, it transports the decomposed materials through the blood to the liver and kidneys. It is these waste products from the proteins that render the body fluids more acid.)

TEN

OSCAR, OUR PET-SQUIRREL.

HERE IS A real life example from my own back yard that may help you better understand the practice of what we have been talking about so far.

Allow me to introduce you to Oscar our pet squirrel and his mom, Agnes.

One Saturday morning as I chopped down one of the palm trees in my yard that had grown too close to the house, I noticed a squirrel running away from the falling tree and jumping into the a tree nearby, squeaking and whipping her tail at us. In the top of the fallen tree I found a squirrel nest with three baby squirrels. My daughter who was helping me saw them too. Immediately her mother instinct kicked in. She took the babies under her care and raised them up to full grown squirrels. Every time she would come home from school the squirrels would rush up to her legs and climb on her shoulders and sit there as if she was their mom. She kept one of the squirrels as a pet: Oscar, and took the other two and released them in the woods nearby.

Back to Agnes the mother squirrel. For several hours that day Agnes kept squeaking and acting very upset, but by the end of the day we did not hear her anymore. She had given up her babies and went on with her life, having to take care of food and shelter for herself for the next days.

When I chopped down Agnes's nest and separated her from her babies, something happened in her breasts. Her milk glands had been producing milk for her three kids right up to the time of the tree falling. Her breasts must have been full of milk and now suddenly her babies were gone! A painful disaster, I'm sure! But here nature came to her rescue.

Because of the sudden shock of the separation, Agnes's nervous system, sensing the emotional turmoil, directed sudden death to the cells in the lining of the milk tubes in her breast.

And because of the widening of the ducts in her breasts milk could flow and the pressure in her breasts could slowly come down to normal. The process may have taken a few days at the most. I hope you see how wonderfully this shows the cooperation and integration of all the physical functions, working together to tackle a serious problem and bring everything back again to the normal way of functioning, to rest.

When Agnes was deprived of her babies, her emotions were soaring, her kids were taken away, her nest was demolished, her breasts were hurting, where would she sleep and take cover for the predators, etc. etc.?

In this moment of panic nature provided the proper response. Agnes's emotions triggered her brain to come with a quick solution to her milk pile up and the pain of her exploding breasts. The milk duct area of the brain got involved (target mark!) and directed the ductal tissue to shed the inner lining of the ducts to give way to the over-abundance of milk to flow to the nipple and relieve the breasts of their load.

What a relieve!

This meaningful process lasted several hours to maybe a day or two. And then...it stopped, because Agnes pulled herself out of her panic mode. She had to 'suck it up' and go on with her life; she needed a new shelter in a new tree while trying to keep all sorts of predators away.

Agnes simply did not have time to allow herself to carry on with her emotions. She had to wipe her emotional slate clean and live on without looking backwards. Nature insisted on it. So when her emotional brain came to rest, there was no further trigger to the brain to provide for better milk flow in the ducts and the ductal cell death program came to a halt. It never developed into full blown ductal cancer of the breasts because she came quickly to resolution of her conflict. And that is the most important lesson we can learn from this animal case history.

It is the continuation of our emotional conflicts, fears, worries, for days and weeks and months that causes a totally good, meaningful, and functional healing program to continue on for too long and to cause the problem we call: cancer.

It is with every manifestation of cancer that we will find this prolonged worry, or this continuing fear, or this unstopped self-devaluation, the everlasting feeling of abandonment, the lasting feeling of our world collapsing, etc., etc. Emotions that we allow to drag on in our lives.

Our emotions were meant to quickly alert us to danger and to guide us to safety, or to redirect us, or stop us in our tracks. We were not designed to be depressed, or fearful, or to worry for days and weeks and months at a time. But when we hang on to our emotions, our beautifully functional system continues to respond to our feelings of fear, worry, or separation by over-reacting, over-assisting, over-healing. Animals are quick to get over their hang-ups, fears, worries and conflicts. Nature offers them no time to linger, meditate, contemplate or dwell on a problem or conflict. The emotional shocks and physical responses that we have talked about are quickly dealt with in nature.

It is our human nature that tends to take its sweet time in digesting our problems and worries. The reason for this is that we have feelings. So where Oscar's mom walked away from her loss of her babies, we tend to be absorbed and over-taken by the feelings that come with the conflict, causing us to take weeks and months to get over our anxiety, sadness, conflict and issues.

An important thing to realize, is that we humans have the ability to not only suffer from an emotional shock in a direct or literal sense; we can also suffer a conflict in a figurative or metaphorical sense.

For instance, although there may not be a real and physical separation going on in a marriage, each of the partners can suffer separation conflicts when they <u>feel</u> that the partner has left them.

Or, the worry for a child can be totally illogical since the child gets all it needs from loving foster parents, or from the nurses in a hospital. Still the mother worries continually for the child's wellbeing because of her <u>feelings</u> of not being able to be there herself.

It is our feelings that can keep us in an emotional strangle hold with the rogue consequence of turning a functional healing process into full blown cancer!

Let's do a quick review of this chapter.

We've looked at the two phases of cancer and the two types of breast cancer; glandular and ductal cancer. Both cancers start off as perfectly normal and meaningful biological healing processes, triggered by a sudden, unexpected and emotional shock to the system.

When the emotional shock is not resolved these processes continue on and eventually create tumors or ulcers (holes). Now it is called cancer.

When the shock is resolved, the woman is transferred into the healing phase of cancer where the cancer activity is stopped. In the healing phase the damage is restored by the body itself: where there is a tumor it dies off and where there is loss of tissue (a hole) there is growth and filling in of new tissue.

Animals also have a physical response after an emotional jolt. However, because of their quick emotional turnaround, cancer is hardly seen.

We humans hold on to our emotions and our feelings for too long and because of this, cancer has a greater chance with us.

We have discussed the two phases of the cancer process. Just like the tide moving in and out we can see the physical programs of our body coming to the aid of our tissues and then retract again, in and out, active and passive, and most of the time we will never become aware of the healings taking place in even the most remote parts of our body. It is only when our feelings keep us in an emotional "cramp' that these meaningful processes become over-abundant. It is often at that moment of an overflowing healing response that we start calling the process: cancer. Before that moment all is well with our body and we reap the great benefits from the meaningful programs our system provides for us.

In our present medical culture cancer may be regarded as a terrible enemy. However, it is we who are forcing our perfect body to continue to heal because of our over-loaded emotional brain, filled with the unresolved feelings that we seem to have so little control over.

What a simple but deep truth and how grateful we can be to Dr. Hamer, who has gone the extra mile to hand us this gift of understanding that cancer is caused and triggered by our own feelings and emotions. We can truly be grateful because we can now take this truth and apply it to our lives and the lives of our loved ones to become whole again without having to use all the monstrosities of the present medical system.

There is no further need for fear, panic, anxiety and death because we have found the cause of cancer. It is within ourselves and we know now what to do!

Or, relating to the parable of the water coming down the stairs, we now know where to find the tap and how to close it even before the water starts to overflow the bath tub.

Eleven

TWO CASE STORIES

Let's have some fun and do a couple of practical case studies to teach you how to deal with cancer in your own body and how to help your friends and family.

Jacky is called a health freak by her friends. She is a 40 year old teacher in high school and in her free time she visits any and every meeting about health she can go to. Jacky is a raving vegetarian. She has read too many books about health. Practices yoga; plays volleyball on the beach and swims laps every morning. She is married to Ben who is a mechanic in the air force, having to work at times out of the country for months at a time. There is not much time for them to talk about more than the necessary stuff. Ben, 44 years old, has been working in Alaska for three months. At his last medical checkup the doc had told him to start with medication because his blood pressure was way too high. Ben ignored the whole matter and when he left, Jacky had a bad feeling that something would happen to him. She was and still is very worried about Ben's wellbeing. Her mother died of a stroke caused by high blood pressure.

After her yearly mammogram Jacky gets a phone call from her doctor and makes an appointment. Doc tells her she has the beginning of a lump in her right breast and she needs to have more X-rays taken and see a specialist.

Driving home Jacky loses it. She is panic stricken and she is furious. - *"I cannot have cancer! I have done everything to stay healthy, I am healthy, I cannot have cancer!"*-, she yells as she hits her fists at the steering wheel. When she gets home she calls Deb her friend, who walks over to her house. Deb knows her stuff; she knows about Doctor Hamer. After Jacky spewed most of her anger and fear to Deb, Deb takes charge and sits her down at the kitchen table. She explains some of Dr. Hamer's ideas to Jacky, who calms down and lends her a listening ear. *"Which breast is involved?"* she asks Jacky. It is her right breast, and knowing that Jacky is right handed gives Deb already some valuable information. *"Have you asked the doctor in what specific tissue you have the lump?"* Jacky did not ask the doctor, she was too overwhelmed by the bad news. Deb instructs her to make an immediate appointment with the specialist and insists that she asks him about the kind of tissue the lump is in.

Five days later they sit at the kitchen table again. *'What did he tell you?"* Deb wants to know. Jacky wrote down what the specialist told her: - adenoid mammary carcinoma -. *"Cancer in your breast gland!"*, says Deb while she reaches in her tote bag and pulls out a large chart and a book and puts them on the table.

"This is Dr. Hamer's chart. Let's look up what the cause is of your cancer and how to get rid of it."

Deb has Jacky's complete attention and in 15 minutes Deb guides Jacky through the book and the chart. Here is what they find: Since Jacky is **right handed** and her **right breast** is involved with a cancer of the **glandular tissue** they already have a wealth of information. Since Jacky deals with glandular cancer they know that it is a **worry conflict** that started the whole thing. And they know that the worry is related to her **husband**. (Right breast – right handed) Deb asks Jacky: *"so what's going on between you and Ben? You want to tell me? What are you so worried about?"*

Jacky goes wide open and tells Deb that she has been having Ben on her mind day and night. She is worried sick about him working too hard and getting a stroke.

"Bingo!" sings Deb, *"that's it, that's it!"*

In another fifteen minutes Deb explains to Jacky Dr. Hamer's ideas of the cause of her breast cancer. It is her worry for Ben that started the whole thing and both realize now how important it will be that Jacky gets over her worry. They talk until late that night and Deb makes sure that Jacky expresses any worry and fear that is still in her heart. They pray about it and take time to intercede for Ben's health and blood pressure. The next day Deb calls Ben in Alaska and tells him how important it will be to take away Jacky's fear and worry for his health issues. Later that day Ben calls Jacky unexpectedly and tells her the good news that his blood pressure has been running lower in the last two weeks. (Of course he thought it wasn't important enough to call her about!)

Jacky starts to sleep better and she does not wake up every two hours anymore. Her shivers are gone and her hands and feet feel warm again. Her worry for Ben has subsided. At the next check-up with the oncologist he tells her that the lump in her breast has not grown any larger. The growth of her cancer had stopped. Jacky realizes that she is now in the healing phase.

DEBBIE'S STORY:

Jacky's friend Debby (Deb) discovered Dr.Hamer's material during her own struggle with cancer five years ago. She went through a painful separation after she found that her husband Anthony had become too friendly with a girl from work and spent his afterhours with her instead of coming home from work. The divorce was fast and complete. He left her to live with the girl in another state. The whole matter had hit Debby like a freight train. In one month time she was back to living on her own in a large and half-empty house. Emotionally she was ravaged, having no one to really share her heart with.

Three months later. Unexpectedly she was called by the doctor after her yearly mammogram. -*"It looks cancerous"*- he said. She did not panic, there was no fear; she was still too stunned by her feeling of loneliness, separated from her Anthony.

After coming home she spent a whole day doing research on the Internet about alternative cancer treatments. She wrote down everything she felt was of value to her. The next day Debby looked at some You-tube videos explaining breast cancer from Dr. Hamer's point of view. After listening multiple times and making notes, Debby knew that this doctor was talking right into her own situation; she wrote down: *- I am **left handed** with cancer in my **left breast**. My left breast is my 'partner breast'. I have cancer in my ducts (**ductal cancer**, said the oncologist), which is caused by a 'separation conflict'. I am a divorcee and I have been left by "the Jerk" (you guessed it: Anthony). Ergo: I have cancer because the Jerk left me and my emotions have gotten the best and, in my case, the worst of me.-*

It took another two days for Deb to understand and admit that her cancer had not started because of the Jerk, **but because of how she emotionally responded to his leaving**.

Harboring resentment and hatred only fired up her feelings of being lonely and miserable, which would prolong the growing of cancer in her breast. She had to forgive and forget in order to start looking forward and drop that feeling of loneliness.

Prayer did a lot for her; she emptied her heart to God and found a renewed relation with Him that filled up the emptiness in her.

The purchase of 'Whiskers', her new Siamese cat, proved to be an excellent choice to redirect her attention and to fill in some of the lonely moments.

At the next visit to the oncologist Debby heard that, just as with Jacky, her cancer had stopped growing. By resolving the emotional shock of the separation there was no further need for her cancer and she too moved into the healing phase.

Twelve

DO THE MATH! FOUR QUESTIONS.

So, HOPEFULLY YOU have a better idea now of what to do when your doc tells you that you have cancer?
Ask yourself the following questions:
1. Which breast is involved; left or right?
2. Am I left or right handed? (When in doubt use the clap test.)
3. Which kind of tissue is involved? Ductal or glandular tissue? Ask your doctor!
4. When did the cancer start? Again; ask your doctor.

As you have seen in the above cases, you do not need to panic or freak out. You just need to know a few things and put two and two together.

Now you can establish what the **cause** is of your cancer. For instance: it's the left breast. I am right handed. (So this is my nest side: my children!) The cancer is found in the glandular tissue. (Worry about somebody in my 'nest') It started approximately two months ago (Aha, this is the time my daughter Allison left for college!)

Yes, this is the time I started worrying about her being with all these other girls and, especially, boys. I called her every day. I began to sleep interrupted. I now remember this was the time I started to have these cold hands and feet and waking up too early in the morning, worrying about Allison.

When you know all this, you have found the answer to your question: - *"why do I have cancer?"* -. You have a worry conflict about your daughter going to college for the first time! Your emotions and feelings of worry for your daughter fire on the milk glands in your left breast to better care for your daughter. (Nature's way of caring is providing more nutrition; milk!)

It's up to you to stop all this by resolving the worry for your daughter. You need to *"get over it"*. And fast! And when you do, **your cancer stops growing** and you will transfer into the healing phase where you'll start to feel different: you will sleep better and longer again, your appetite will pick up, you'll feel warm again, etc. and the cancerous lump will literally die and shrivel up.

THIRTEEN

BACK TO: CANCER IN AMERICA

WE NEED TO step back for a moment into the reality of the *'run-off-the-mill'* breast cancer treatments in America anno 2014. Most women detect their breast cancer at the moment they have transferred into the healing phase, simply because this is the time the breast starts hurting and, or, swelling. The pain and swelling direct the women to do a self-exam and when they feel something suspicious they will make an appointment to visit the doctor. The doctor also examines and makes X-rays and will send them to the specialist for treatment of the cancer. Most likely you will not find a doctor in your town that is proficient in the principles of Germanic New Medicine and the ideas of Dr. Hamer. The doctor who has detected your breast cancer has likely never heard of a conflict active phase and a healing phase, as suggested by Dr. Hamer. And you, very likely, will not convince him to change his course of treatment by having him read this book.

He will steer you into the treatment direction of *'consensus medicine'*, which is: the general accepted treatment that is also being done by all his peers and colleagues: taking a biopsy, doing chemo-treatment, radiation and, if needed, surgery of the breast.

Now you will have to make a choice:

You either stay on your course with GNM, knowing that you already are in the healing phase and that your cancer has stopped growing. It may take quite a while; you will feel like sleeping a lot, there may be swelling, bacteria, temperature and pain, but your body will eventually clean up the tumor, or the ulceration, all by itself if you give your body what it needs: rest and proper nutrition.

Or, you go with the oncologist's plan, in which case you will be given chemicals that were created to kill all fast growing cells in your body. The chemo- treatment will hopefully kill all the cancer cells, but in the process will also kill many of your normal, healthy cells. (<u>Now remember; when you are in the healing phase, the cancer cells are already dying, even without any treatment.</u>)

This chemo-treatment may give you the mother of all hangovers. Vomiting, diarrhea, dizziness, nausea, loss of taste, loss of sleep and appetite, muscle weakness, loss of balance, your hair may fall out, etc. and you may have to do repeated treatments to - *'make sure we got it all'* -.

You may be lucky and have only a few of these symptoms.

But wait; there is more. After the chemo treatment there is possibly radiation treatment, where the cancer cells, plus some of the surrounding tissue, simply are burned to death. Both these treatments can have horrendous side effects. Surgery may even be suggested and you possibly may lose one or both of your breasts and more...

The choice is yours of course. And I realize and acknowledge that, although it may look easy on paper, it will take a lot of guts to follow a course where you will be ridiculed and not understood. You will be called stupid, pig headed, suicidal and what not, because you are going against the grain.

However you will also blaze a trail for the women around you, who are panic stricken by the thought of getting breast cancer. You will be one of the first women in your area who will lead the way out of a medical culture where women have their breasts amputated out of fear.

But you're not the only one. More women have gone the course of Dr. Hamer with good success. You can read about some of them on the website of Dr. C. Markolin: www.learninggnm.com and then look under 'Therapy' and 'Testimonials'.

In his bio, at the end of this book, you will find that Dr. Hamer's success rate is 90+ percent.

Fourteen

QUESTIONS & ANSWERS

METASTASIS; CAN CANCER SPREAD FROM ONE TISSUE TO ANOTHER?

WOMEN, WHO ARE not familiar with the principles of GNM and who have never heard of cancer being caused by sudden emotional shocks, fears or worries can be exposed to yet another set of challenges triggered by the conventional treatments themselves.

Let me explain. So far we have only been talking about breast cancer. However, according to GNM, not just breast cancer but **all** cancers are started by specific emotional shocks, fears, and worries. And while going through conventional treatment, with its horrible side-effects, a woman may be very vulnerable for even more emotional turmoil, which can be the cause for more and different types of cancers.

For instance, lung cancer is triggered by the *fear of death*. Bone-, muscle- and lymph-node cancer is caused by *'self-devaluation' conflicts*.

It does not take much imagination to see how a woman, who hears from her doctor that she has stage three breast cancer, may also start cancer in the lung right at that moment caused by a **sudden fear of death** in the doctor's office.

Or lymph node cancer, which is the result of a *self-devaluation conflict*, is often seen in combination with breast cancer. We can imagine a women's fear of disfigurement before a future breast surgery and the drop in feeling of self-worth this may lead to.

All these emotional conflicts can each express themselves in a (new) form of cancer in the neighboring tissues of the breast; the ribs (bone tissue), the muscles between the ribs, the lymph nodes close to the breast, or the lung tissue under the breast.

It is understandable that these new expressions of cancer, in the vicinity of the cancerous breast, may give the impression that the cancer in the breast is spreading. This has formed the basis for the <u>theory of</u> '*metastasis*', or 'the spreading of cancer', that has become dogma in the medical community.

The theory of metastasis, however, is still a theory and has never been proven. There are several counter arguments that make the whole idea of metastasis impossible.

For instance: if individual 'malignant' cancer cells would travel through the body, they would do this by means of the blood or the lymph fluid. Well, cancer cells are not found in lymph fluid or in the blood stream. And if they would be found in the blood, we can be sure that every blood donor would have to be screened for cancer before giving blood, right?

And they're not.

IS CANCER A GENETIC DISEASE?

In America the subject of genes has become a big issue in the discussion on cancer. The idea that you can have cancer-genes can hang over your head as a ton of bricks. In these last years this is driving women to where they have their breasts surgically removed, probably because they are tired of living with the constant fear that their genes can start the fire of cancer any time and at any place.

So, is it the genes making me more of a candidate for cancer than other people?

Well, apparently, there are genes that have the potential to do just that, and when these genes were discovered they became the talk of the town for a while and many believed in the inevitability of the genetic cause of cancer. Genes were it and when you had them, you were doomed!

Now, wooh, wooh, not so fast...!

In GNM thinking we do not want to call these genes '*cancer-genes*'. Remember, we only talk about cancer after a special biological program continues on for longer than it was intended! So, although the genes may play an initial role in starting a special (healing) program, we should not blame them for carrying on with the program for too long. That is not their fault! It is caused by the owner of the genes!

Also, in the last ten years a new science has found its place in the discussion about genes. It is called 'epigenetics'; studying the influence of the environment of the cell on the expression of the cell's genes.

Although the DNA in the gene gives a gene its *potential* to express cancer, it does not have the first or final say in this matter. Through the epigenetic approach, it is found more and more that the *expression* of (cancer) genes is very much dependent on what is happening or not happening in the influence sphere (the milieu) around the cell.

This cell milieu is like a soup where the cell floats in together with literally thousands of other chemical structures that all convey very specific messages to the cell.

Lynne McTaggart is an investigative journalist and author of several interesting books about cutting edge information on what is happening in the wonderful world of science. In her latest book: "the Bond" (2012, Free Press) she writes on page 24:

-"*The intricate array of **environmental influences** to which we are exposed throughout our lives **actually determines the final expression of every gene in our body**. Genes get turned on, turned off, or modified by our life circumstances and environment: what we eat, who we surround ourselves with, and how we lead our lives.*"

And a little further: -*"Epigenetic changes and the ultimate expression or silencing of a gene occur as a result of environmental stressors. Diet, the quality of air and water,* **the emotional climate** *within your family, the state of your relationships, your sense of fulfillment in life – the sum total of how you live your life and also how your ancestors lived theirs - have the most effect on the expression of your genes."*

Genes do not have the final say! I repeat the above: - *"the sum total of how you live your life has the most effect on the expression of your genes."* -

How we live our life, the choices we make on a daily base, the worry we allow ourselves, the fears we grew up with, they all matter and they all have their influence on the genes in these tiny little cells that our tissues consist of.

And so how can we prevent cancer? How do we keep our genes from being influenced negatively by our emotions?

PREVENTION OF CANCER

Germanic New Medicine has paved the way for us to finally understand the cause and trigger of breast cancer. The sudden, unexpected conflict, fear, or worry is the trigger for every cancer in the body. Of course this does not mean that every worry, fear or conflict will result in cancer! Many people have been hit in their life by severe emotional shocks, worries and fears that never resulted in any kind of cancer, while other people seem to be prone to contracting cancer more than others. Why are some people so prone to cancer? The reason for this is unknown.

However, in GNM we now have found the way to stop cancer in its tracks!

Let me explain and let's follow Dr. Hamer's (GNM's) thought pattern.

When the growth of glandular cells is triggered in the breast after a sudden worry, we have learned that this is a '*special and meaningful biological program'* and that this program will continue as long as the psyche / spirit is 'engaged' in this worry.

The spirit choses a plan to relieve this worry and communicate this plan to the brain. The brain acts like the contractor and directs the work that is being done at the work site: the breast. And we have seen that this dynamic continues as long as the spirit / psyche is being engaged in this worry.

We also have learned about the physical signs indicating that we are in the conflict active phase.

When the worry has been resolved within, let's say, three weeks, the woman probably will never have noticed that anything went on in her breast. But when she stays engaged in this worry, the program will continue to grow glandular cells until she or her doctor finds a lump in her breast. Now we are talking about cancer.

I hope you see now that when we take the worry out of this equation, the special and meaningful biological program is stopped at the right time because there is no further need for the program to continue and end in cancer.

So, yes, we can prevent breast cancer, by recognizing that we are in the conflict active phase and by resolving our worry conflict (glandular), or our separation conflict (ductal) as soon as possible.

HOW TO RESOLVE STUBBORN AND PERSISTENT EMOTIONAL ISSUES

First of all, we should be able to deal with issues simply around the kitchen table. When you have detected that you have an issue pressing on your heart and conscience, which prevents you from having a normal healthy sleep, do not immediately presume that you have cancer! Chances are that you just have to work through an issue that you are upset about and that may 'evaporate' in a few days. No big deal, we all go through them almost daily.

It is, however, a good life-strategy to live with a clean conscience and without any issues. It is do-able and highly recommended.

"Don't worry, be happy!"

When we hold on to issues, worries, fears, anger, etc. they all pile up in our emotional brain, or Mid-brain, which is hard wired, by the nerves, to our body tissues (our muscles, glands, etc.).

The Mid-brain files and stores every experience that has triggered a negative emotion or feeling in the history of a person. It does this so we can anticipate danger, and to get us ready for action; either to fight and defend ourselves, or to make a run for it.

When one of these negative feelings or emotions is re-activated by a new, related, experience, many switches are being flipped causing all sorts of physical changes.

You can imagine that when these negative emotions are not dealt with, they can accumulate to where we are easily overcome by an over loaded Mid-brain that continually triggers our body with stress signals. (High blood pressure, high sugar, and adrenaline in the blood stream, poor appetite and sleep, etc.)

So let's deal with them.

Here are some suggestions:

- Take the time to listen to your heart! Really listen...! No TV, cell-phone, face-book.

- Open your heart; be transparent and talk to someone you trust. A good friend or family member. By talking about the issue you deflate the presence of it in the Mid-brain.

- I highly recommend talking to God about the things inside your heart, because often you don't even know what is in there and He does; He is an expert! Asking His Holy Spirit to reveal what is in your heart may lead to some surprising moments. I have had many immediate answers on my own questions.

- Sometimes you have dealt with an issue that just doesn't want to leave and let go. Like a piece of duct tape that keeps sticking to your finger. You cannot get rid of and the issue keeps bouncing around in your head.

    An excellent technique to relieve this is EFT, or Emotional

Freedom Technique. A simple way of tapping with your fingers on acupuncture points on your body while speaking out what is bugging you. You will find a description in my other book: "Away with Cancer", or you can find the manual for EFT on the Internet at numerous web-sites. EFT has proven to be one of the best ways to relieve Post Traumatic Stress Syndrome in war veterans. This is a simple technique you can learn in 10 minutes and have a friend for life. Try www.emofree.com.

- As I am writing these last pages I came across a book that deals with emotions that somehow have become trapped during our busy lives.
  I can recommend the book: '*The Emotion Code*', by author Dr. Bradley Nelson. He gives you 'do it yourself' instructions for uncovering these emotions and he teaches you how to release and eliminate them.

WHAT ABOUT ALTERNATIVE TREATMENTS?

Herbs, minerals, vitamins, potions, salves, fruits, vegetables, rain forest fruits, bee pollen and tree-bark have proven to be formidable cancer fighters for those who have used them. I have written a book about them (Away with Cancer) and feel passionate about the many ways these natural, God given substances have helped people in their search for health.

The great difference with Dr. Hamer's ideas is that most of these above mentioned substances are used by people to...*fight* cancer and with the aim to kill cancer cells.

I hope you have discovered that, now that you know the cause of cancer, with GNM you are learning to...*heal* cancer by taking away the cause of cancer!

This is an entirely different approach.

Too often I talk with well-meaning people who, in their attempt to kill cancer, are using a two barreled shotgun filled with as much substances they can afford, shooting in random at anything they see moving.

My heart goes out to them and I feel a great sense of belonging with this band of folks who have seen and often experienced the devastation of "cancer treatment" and have decided to *'walk it alone'* and *'go natural'*.

I have written this book mostly for them. They, most of all, deserve to know that healing from cancer is possible and I am confident that they will carry Dr. Hamer's message of hope to those who need it.

EARTHING?

Earthing; what on earth is that?

Well, earthing is kind of a new term used for making electrical contact with the earth by, for instance, taking off your shoes and walking on the wet beach, or a wet lawn or dirt-road. By doing this we allow our bodies to be replenished with electrons from the earth.

As you know we are all basically electrical beings, held together by the continual exchange of electrical particles and charges. Since the fifties people have been walking on shoes with rubber soles that insulate us from the earth and that prevent us from getting our daily supply of healthy electrons from the earth.

Research is being done about earthing and so far there seems to be a relation between our lack of daily electrons and the state of disease our western culture is in. For instance, a simple test was done of looking through a microscope at a drop of live blood. The blood plates can be seen moving around. In diseased people the platelets are often clumped together, but when a diabetic patient was connected for 2 hours with an earth-connected wire, his blood plates reacted quite differently: they were moving around freely and not being clumped together, which is a sign of good health!

A new industry is on the rise fabricating and marketing different ways of reconnecting with the earth, like foot pads and special bed-sheets that connect you with the earth by the earth cable of your house.

In a previous page the question came up of why we have become so vulnerable to all sorts of diseases, among which cancer.

Could it be that since we have become insulated from the normal natural flow of healthy electrons, we are missing a key ingredient in the normal health maintenance of our bodies?

And let's go a step further; since diseases and especially cancer, are so linked to our emotional well-being, could it be that we are experiencing in our emotional brain the detrimental effects of a "low battery", or a lack of ability to "discharge"?

Please try this out for yourself and if you cannot walk on the beach, try walking with your bare feet on the wet grass after the rain.

The book 'Earthing' has as subtitle: - *the most important health discovery ever?* –

It may very well be!

WHAT ABOUT PRAYER?

I whole heartedly believe in praying for the sick in church, or at home, or at the kitchen table. Most of us know people who were healed by the power that God gives when there are people praying. The God of Abraham, Isaac and Jacob, as He wants to be known, is a good God, full of compassion for us.

Still, even in our churches, many people succumb to diseases and are not healed. We'll have to be open and honest about this. This should be a great frustration of any Christian; we are not seeing a breakthrough in the battle against cancer and against disease in general.

The only conclusion we must draw from this situation is that we are doing something wrong! But, what?

That small question has been and still is the focus of many of my prayer walks. What, pray tell, do we do wrong? What do we not see, or do we see wrongly? Why do we not see more healing as an answer to prayer, while it was Jesus himself who told us that we will do more and greater things than He did?

Although I do not have a satisfying answer as of yet, I do believe that an answer must be found in our attitude towards, again, the treatment of disease.

Growing up in our Western culture, we have learned to put our full trust in the authority of white coated men or women, who have a degree in the pharmaceutical (= chemical) approach to the treatment of disease.

These doctors are bound to practice "consensus medicine", which is the preferred treatment protocol that is approved and protected by an enormous body of corporate and political interests, that finds its existence in the making of money and in wielding an unrighteous control over its market and the people in that market.

This market forbids and condemns the real research for the cause of cancer.

In this market there is no room for health, healing or a cure for disease, because health is regarded as the competitor of treatment that keeps the system from generating more profit.

In the Bible this system is called the Mammon, a system opposed to the Kingdom of God.

We can have respect for medical professionals who do the best they can for their patients and we may count ourselves blessed by being able to buy medication, if we would need some; however we have sold our soul to this system if we have given up our quest to find the cause of disease in general and of cancer in particular.

In this attitude we are not on God's side and we may not be under His protection.

This is why Dr. Hamer's ideas are of such monumental importance for our Western culture, not only in the way we look at cancer but moreover in our attitude towards all diseases! In GNM we can re-find what has been kept from us for so long: the simple cause of our sickness. And we can find it where it has been for all this time: within ourselves!

The Cause and Cure of Breast Cancer

This simple but so profound truth gives us back our response-ability to keep our good health, and it gives us back the power to recover from disease.

GNM also re-opens the curtains that were pulled closed to the Creator.

In our culture God is often portrayed as a capricious god, smiting people left and right with the most horrendous suffering, using our physical bodies as receptacles for his wrath.

GNM gives us new vision and understanding that what we have called disease is not an enemy, but in principle a very meaningful healing response, originating in our spirit, directed by our brain and executed by our tissues, in answer to a threat, a fear, a worry or a conflict.

What a God-given system. How well created!

And we can control all this simply by resolving our emotional conflicts within the right time frame and to make sure we never hold a grudge to anyone.

Well, so, what about prayer?!

With the new system of GNM we now can pray with greater clarity, vision, hope, direction and faith. Since we have learned what causes cancer, we can ask the Holy Spirit more *specifically* about:

- ✓ what conflict ignited the cancer,
- ✓ revelation about the conflict, fear or worry,
- ✓ why am I so vulnerable for these conflicts,
- ✓ what is the underlying cause of my fear,
- ✓ how can I overcome my worry,
- ✓ help, support, strength and guidance in the healing phase.
- ✓ etc., etc.

And when we have new vision and understanding of the cause and the course of a disease like breast cancer, we have no more reason to be afraid.

Cancer does not scare us anymore!

We can have good faith and trust that even if cancer would be found in our tissues, we now have the know-how to reverse it in due time.

And lastly, prayer by itself does not have to mean the constant and repetitious request for healing. After asking for the healing we are also commanded to exercise our trust and faith.

I have made it a habit, after asking for anything, to start thanking for God's provision.

CONCLUSION

I HOPE I KEPT my promise of keeping the size of this booklet down to where you can carry it around in your purse.

I did that for a good reason. When you have read and understood the material in this book, you have become a life saver for your female friends and family members. What is easier than to whip this booklet out any time you talk with them about breast cancer around the kitchen table, or at your kids' soccer practice. You have answers. You now know the cause of breast cancer.

While the cancer treatment mills are turning at top speed, you now have a good reason to simply stay out of their reach because...*you know better*!

What a blessing to live without the fear of cancer! And what a blessing you can be to all those around you that still live in fear, because they do not yet know the true dynamics and cause of cancer.

How instrumental you can become in the lives of people with this simple but helpful knowledge.

Be like a bra to them; close to their heart and always there for support! Have an extra copy in your purse.

Dr. Hamer has given us clear understanding of the cause of cancer. I have found that his insight finally has completed my own idea of the existence of disease and cancer. I always knew in my spirit that cancer is strongly related to the things that are going on in the core of our being; our heart and our emotions. In my practice I have seen it in most of my patients.

God has not given us a body full of trapdoors and land mines that can go off at any given time, as we are told to believe. He has created us very well and the special and meaningful biological programs that run in response to our emotional well, or not-so-well-being, are true gifts of Him to keep us healthy and to respond adequately to the challenges of our busy environment.

Our genes are not the capricious instigators of mayhem, as we are told, that can start a fire in our bodies at any time. God is still Master of His universe and the Creator of our bodies, giving us the task of being good stewards over our emotional and physical domain.

It is our job to keep our Mid-brain, our heart, or core as clean as we can. And although we often cannot prevent the daily challenges that living in our culture brings with it, we will have to keep short accounts with the things that upset us in order to maintain our health.

The apostle Paul writes in the Bible to not go asleep while still being angry. It is a principle that, I believe, not only works when being angry, but with any emotional challenge, conflict, fear and worry that comes our way.

And what better way to live with a clear conscience and Mid-brain then to live a transparent life! We were not meant to live as individuals on our own islands in the ocean of our western culture. We were meant to have heart to heart relationships, sharing each other's ups and downs.

Another principle worthy of mentioning here is that of forgiveness. It is curious to find that not only the bible, but even many scientific writings of the last decennia warn us not only to always forgive, but to do it...immediately.

In the parable of Jesus in Matthew 18 of the 'unforgiving servant', a heavy consequence is carried by those who do not forgive:...physical *torture*!

So put this book in your purse and be a force for good!

Now go and win this fight!

God bless you.

I WANT TO ENCOURAGE the reader to take time and go to the website of Caroline Markolin Ph D.: www.learninggnm.com

She is a student of Dr. Hamer and a wonderful teacher; she teaches GNM on her website and on several Youtube video's. I cannot praise her enough for her talent in teaching the difficult material of GNM and make it understandable.

DR. HAMER'S BIO

For those of you who may wonder what happened to Dr. Hamer, I recommend that you read his biography that was written by Dr. Caroline Markolin Ph D., who did a more than excellent job in describing the very hard road that Dr. Hamer (born in 1935) has travelled in his lifetime.

It would take half of this book to describe the vicious attacks on Dr. Hamer's ideas and work as well as on his personal life and how it affected his practice.

The powers that be prove themselves over and over again to be deathly afraid that the truth of German New Medicine will reach the general public and that it will take off the blinds of the professionals in the medical community.

The University of Tuebingen (Germany) so far has refused to even look into Dr. Hamer's material and, to add insult to injury, has given him an ultimatum to deny his findings and to change his mind, or else...

More than once Dr. Hamer has seen jail cells from the inside and in different countries.

For us it is good to know that, in preparing their court case against Dr. Hamer, his opponents looked up 6500 of Dr. Hamer's old cancer patients, hoping to be able to give documented substance to their case. To their surprise and disgust however, they found 6000 of his patients, whom Dr. Hamer had treated for cancer, still in good health.

They proved Dr. Hamer had a cancer cure-rate of 90%, which is unheard of in our medical culture!

APPENDIX

We always learn most from people who can say: "*been there and done that*". Here are four testimonies from women who were healed from breast cancer while following Dr. Hamer's teachings. Dr. Markolin graciously allowed these testimonies to be extracted from her website and used in this book.

"WE THANK GNM FOR A NEW LIFE!"

This is the story of my former companion, who was cured of breast cancer through German New Medicine. To keep it simple, I will refer to her in this account as my wife: It was May, when my wife noticed a lump in her left breast while doing a breast self-examination. I had already heard about GNM at this point, but was not yet conversant enough to fully apply it.

So we made an appointment at the hospital to see Professor Dr. Dr. W., the oncologist in charge. After the examination and the subsequent biopsy, my wife received the diagnosis: "malignant breast cancer". As to my questions about what was causing the cancer, the doctor responded with "the environment", "family history", "stress", "smoking", etc. Aside from that, he said, we shouldn't ask so many questions, but rather get immediately an appointment for surgery, otherwise my wife will not survive the next four weeks.

I thought of German New Medicine. I phoned the GNM workshop facilitator in X, who is also a practitioner. First of all he calmed us down. Then, he invited us to join the next GNM study group. There, together with others interested in GNM, we were in a setting where we could investigate and discuss the cause of my wife's breast cancer. We quickly established that my wife had suffered a "worry conflict" over her son. The clapping test clearly showed that she is **right-handed**, which is why she developed the breast cancer (glandular) in her *left* **breast**. My wife had a son from her previous marriage, who was drinking excessively. One day, when he was 29 years old, she found him dead in his bed. This was, of course, a tremendous shock for her. The brain CT, obtained shortly after this meeting, confirmed the impact of that conflict-shock. We followed the GNM recommend-dations with full confidence. The next several weeks were entirely dedicated to my wife so that she could come to terms with the conflict.

Solely through the knowledge of GNM - without any conventional medical treatment - within half a year the "malignant" breast tumor eventually had turned into an insignificantly small encapsulated nodule.

We thank GNM for a new life!

For safety reasons, it may be better not to publish my full name. With my very best wishes,

B., January 1, 2009

"WITHIN 4 WEEKS, THE LUMP IN HER BREAST WAS CONSIDERABLY SMALLER"

I have lived mainly in Thailand for the last 18 years and I am married to a Thai lady. Since we were not able to have children ourselves, we had a foster-child with us for just over 7 years. Last year, I had to be in Germany for eight months, which caused a lot of tension between my wife and me. However, this was the only solution, because I had to see to many things in my homeland. Amongst other things, I was finally able to attend a GNM lecture and take part in a seminar. I have been involved with German New Medicine for about four years now and I am thoroughly convinced of it.

About 4 weeks ago, my wife complained about pain in her left breast and let me touch the lump that she had been feeling for a few days. She felt that she had to go to the doctor immediately to get this cleared up. With much patience, I explained to her the Biological Special Program (SBS) of breast cancer and by doing so managed to take away her fear. We then searched our minds for any conflict that could possibly have been responsible for the lump.

Since my wife is right-handed, we knew that it must have been a mother/child conflict. Before my departure for Germany, we had decided that - since my wife's mother had problems with her kidneys - my wife would bring her to our place and help her change her unhealthy eating patterns. This was a huge success, as she was getting better all the time.

However, after a good four months (in September) she decided to go back to her home where she was again exposed to conventional food. My wife was not able to reconcile herself to her mother's decision, and for a time could not bring herself to communicate with her. This was actually the right thing to do, because in that way she could remove herself from the acute conflict and resolve it. It was hardly surprising, therefore, that her symptom would appear by January/February.

Within 4 weeks of our revealing conversation, my wife was noticing that the lump in her breast was considerably smaller, and that the pain had become less within just two weeks. She was ecstatic about this course of events. Today, the lump can hardly be felt anymore, and she trusts entirely that the rest will disappear completely.

It is unimaginable what would have happened, had she turned to conventional medicine (oncology). First she would have had the diagnosis-shock, and then the inevitable "therapy"!

I am infinitely thankful that I came to understand German New Medicine quite well, and have already had the chance to experience the *positive* aspects of that invaluable knowledge. I am sure that GNM will be a considerable part of what is soon going to lead to significant changes in our world, changes towards a more humane future, where materialism will play a subordinate role.

By Hermann Krause, March 14, 2009

"I AM EXCEEDINGLY HAPPY TO KNOW GNM"

It is through my sister-in-law Martina Kloiber, who participated in your GNM seminar in Pocking (Germany) that I heard for the first time about Dr. Hamer's German New Medicine. Since then, this subject has excited me a great deal. It is an incredible discovery!!!

At first, I was irritated when Martina told me about this. But since she described to me in a very trustworthy, serious and "plausible" manner what "German New Medicine" is, I agreed to an 'experiment', meaning a diagnosis according to GNM. In short, I 'buried myself' in your GNM website, studied the material in one quick hurry… and I began to understand how my body functions... I will describe briefly my disease history:

In September 2003, during a 'cancer prevention check-up', a lump was discovered in my right breast.

My doctor scheduled for me, in two days' time, an appointment for a mammogram and he told me that I should quickly proceed with an examination (this took place the same day when I talked to Martina about German New Medicine). The mammogram confirmed: breast cancer!!! At first I didn't want to believe it. That very same day they wanted to do a biopsy to find out whether the tumor was benign or malignant. I declined the biopsy because I wanted to proceed with German New Medicine. It was not easy to free myself from the 'claws' of medical the profession, but I succeeded.

Now I started my 'own' therapy!!! First, I had to identify my conflict...

- I am right-handed
- The lump is in my right breast
- I don't take any medication (not even the pill)
- I have warm hands
- I am not in menopause (age, 42 years)

That means that I had to look for a "partner conflict", but first I couldn't think of any. My relationship was going well and at work everything was also okay at this time. Where should I start looking? And what should I search for?

I screened my life from top to bottom, and then I suddenly found it. My diary helped me realize that in the past I did have problems with my partner, but in reality not WITH but BECAUSE of him.

My partner and I both work in the same branch of a bank, separated by several rooms. One day, a new colleague arrived on the scene, and "she" is a very "pretty blonde"!!! From a professional point of view she is a real ace and for our department a genuine benefit. At first, all went well. But then there were the "awesome" seminars in which my partner and that blonde had to attend. At that time I was on stand-by duty at the office so I wasn't able to attend the seminars with my partner. But when he returned from the seminars he exuberantly described how terrific everything had been. I did not know just what he meant by "terrific". As time went on, I developed a dislike against the other woman. I did not know why - in fact, I really had no reason to be suspicious. But I had that strange feeling.

I knew I had to somehow see clarity in this situation. Despite the fact that I trusted my partner, I thought that maybe he was not capable to resist the charm of that woman. I talked with him about the situation several times and made him understand that I was afraid of losing him. But he always put me at ease and reassured me that all was well. The blonde never found out about my fears. All this persisted for five months and then: SHE moved on and she was gone! She was transferred to another city and told us at the farewell party that soon she would get marry. This took a heavy load off my mind and I was super happy.

The conflict was resolved and now I recognize my track.

In earlier years, I was dumped by my former boyfriend BECAUSE of a blonde woman. I suspect that since then, I always experience a conflict with or because of blonde women.

Back to the history of my disease:

I was conflict active for 5 months (the "other woman" was with us from Jan. 2003 to mid Aug. 2003)

In Sept. 2003, I received the diagnosis of breast cancer (according to conventional medicine)

In Sept. 2003, I learned about German New Medicine

In Jan. 2004, I had another checkup for my breast cancer. The result: no cancer!!!

I am by nature a skeptic. But I have experienced for myself that German New Medicine does not deserve skepticism - only respect and high esteem!

I hope that with your presentations you will be able to open the eyes of many people in this world and make German New Medicine so clear for them that they can escape the insanity of conventional medicine.

I am exceedingly happy to know GNM. With gratitude and best wishes, Silvia Herzig.

PS: What would have happened with my body if I had consented to submit to traditional medicine!? I can only say one thing: Long live German New Medicine!!!

All testimonies were translated from the German original by Caroline Markolin, Ph.D.

Extracted from: http://LearningGNM.com

Disclaimer: The information in these testimonies does not replace professional medical advice.

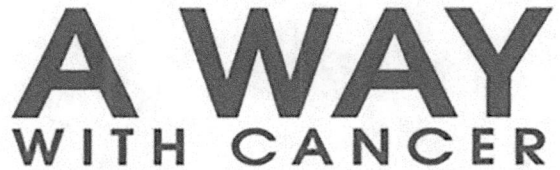

A WAY WITH CANCER

A WAY OUT OF THE CANCER EPIDEMIC

A Cancer Cure Guide
for Serious Do-It-Yourselfers

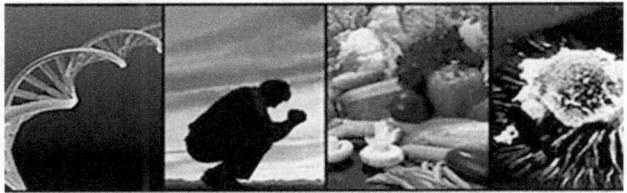

DICK SCHUYT, RPT

Independent researchers have known all along how to prevent, control and cure Cancer, however their results and practical know-how does not reach the general public. This book will change that. Learn how to prevent Cancer and find how others have fought it successfully.

When you like to read more about the reasons why the 'war on cancer' has not been won in spite of the billions of dollars that is spent on research, this book will explain what you need to know. I condensed every alternative treatment for cancer that I was aware of in this book.

260 pages of info about alternative ways to assist your body finding healing and health.

CONTACT

If the information in this book has helped you get well, please let me know your story.

You can contact me by email:

AWAYWITHCANCER@AOL.COM,

or write me at the following address:

**P.O. BOX 144,
ROCKY FACE, GEORGIA, 30740**

For bulk-orders
of "the Cause and Cure of Breast Cancer"
or "Away with Cancer",
write or email me.

www.ingramcontent.com/pod-product-compliance
Lightning Source LLC
Chambersburg PA
CBHW071753170526
45167CB00003B/1009